LIVE
LOVE
LUST

Sadie Cayman

Published by arrangement with Summersdale Publishers Ltd. in the United States by Cleis Press, an imprint of Start Midnight, LLC, 221 River Street, Ninth Floor, Hoboken, New Jersey 07030.

Printed in the United States

10 9 8 7 6 5 4 3 2 1

Trade paper ISBN: 978-1-62778-336-1

E-book ISBN: 978-1-62778-549-5

CONTENTS

INTRODUCTION

Life is for loving. Whatever inspiration you're looking for in your sex life, this book has got you covered. From steamy date night ideas to dirty conversation starters, and from naughty games to raunchy recipes, there will never be another dull moment in your love nest. Flip to the sex facts, positions and tips and you might just learn a new thing or two to impress your lover. If you've got sex on the brain, there are smut-themed wordsearches, crosswords, anagrams and more to keep you satisfied. And if you're a hopeless romantic, there are date night and sex vouchers to tear out and present to your loved one. This book was created for anyone who likes to show their partner a good time—whatever your gender or sexual orientation. Love is love, after all. Let's dive between the covers and get those juices flowing.

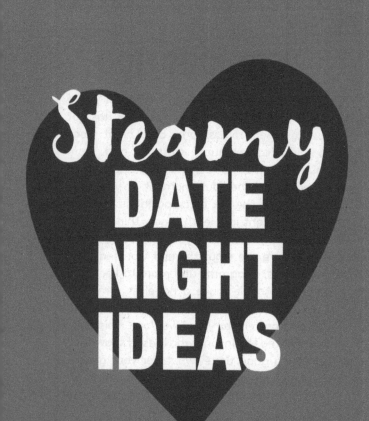

See you in the tub

There's nothing like a long soak in a hot bath to get you feeling relaxed. Why not invite your partner to join you so you can get in the mood together? Light some candles, fill the tub and pop in a luxury bath bomb or some sensual essential oils: try ylang-ylang, jasmine, lavender or cinnamon. Take your time getting undressed for each other. Once you're in, it's time to relax and maybe treat each other to an underwater massage . . . or more. If you don't have a tub, a couple's shower can be just as steamy. Getting your partner lathered up is a great excuse to slowly caress your favorite parts of their body.

Netflix and sizzle

When it's cold outside, why not raise the
temperature with a raunchy movie night
at home with your beau? Pull the curtains,
light some candles and slip into something
comfortable before you begin. Each of you can
select a favorite saucy movie for the evening's
entertainment. Press play and
get cozy as the action unfolds. Take it in
turns to control the remote. When you get
to a sexy scene that turns you on, press pause
and act out the on-screen action
together. The sultry atmosphere combined with
a bit of role-play is bound to set your night on
fire. By the time the credits roll,
you'll be starring in your own sizzler.

Come find me!

Here's a juicy little idea for a date to remember: set up a saucy scavenger hunt by planting clues that will lead them to you. The clues can be in the form of sexy texts or naughty notes—or a combination of both. Lead your partner along a trail, with plenty of cheeky hints as to the pleasures they'll experience when they track you down. Exactly where you lead them is up to you, but here are some options:

 A fancy hotel room that you have booked for a night of fun

 A bar, where they find you in a trench coat with nothing underneath

 Your bedroom, where you lie naked and ready for that thing you've both always wanted to try

Sensual sipping

What could be more classy than an evening enjoying fine wine? Book yourselves on to a wine-tasting session at your local wine bar or winery, or stock up on a selection to try at home. To add an extra layer of full-bodied fun, get a blindfold and take turns guessing which wine you are sampling. The buzz from the wine and the heightened sensation of tasting with your eyes closed are sure to get all those sensory receptors tingling. Remember to sip and not swig. You don't want to end up so inebriated that you aren't able to fully appreciate each other's company by the end of the evening. And keep hold of that blindfold—it could come in handy once you retire to the bedroom . . .

Sultry
spa session

This at-home date is the perfect antidote to the stresses of modern life and will leave you both feeling relaxed and in tune with each other. All you need is a comfortable room, your own fair hands and some massage oil. You could buy an oil blend or try preparing your own by mixing a couple of drops of your favorite essential oil into a carrier oil such as almond, coconut or jojoba. Then give each other a relaxing massage. Communication is key here: be sure to let your partner know when they do something that feels good and tell them which parts of your body you want them to caress and rub.

A trip down memory lane

Remember that special moment when
you realized there was a spark between you?
Recreating your first date at home is a fun way
to recapture what originally brought you
together. If your first date was a dinner, why not
try to reproduce the meal in your own
kitchen? If it was a trip to the movie theater, you
could watch the movie you saw while cuddling
up on your sofa. The romance of it all could
leave you inspired to recreate your first kiss . . .
and other first moments.

Sole mates

Take some time out to pay attention to an often-neglected part of each other's bodies: your feet. Did you know that the soles of the feet have a high concentration of nerve endings, with as many as 200,000 per sole? This makes them supersensitive, and for some people, they are erogenous zones. Whether that's you or not, pampering each other's feet is a sensual way to bond and relax together. Start with foot soaks, maybe throw in a foot detox mask and finish off with foot massages. Tickles are optional.

A night under the stars

Nothing says romance like gazing up at the stars together. On a dry, clear night, roll out the picnic blanket and set up an outdoor feast to enjoy while looking up at the night sky. Drive out to a spot in the countryside away from light pollution. Or, for a home-grown adventure (if you have the space), you could set up a tent in your back garden and camp out together. Cuddling up and getting cozy among the sounds of nature is bound to bring you closer together.

A flirty feast

It's often said that certain foods have aphrodisiac properties. While the scientific evidence to support that may be debatable, seductively feeding each other tasty morsels can be a fun way to get closer and in the mood for pleasure. So, dim the lights, light the candles and serve up a sexy selection of tasty treats. Here are some ideas to get the juices flowing:

 Strawberries (dunked in white chocolate for maximum enjoyment)

 Warmed figs (why not add a squirt of whipped cream?)

 Honey (dab a bit somewhere on your body while your partner's eyes are closed, then challenge them to find it with their tongue)

 Sushi (nyotaimori is often referred to as "body sushi" and is the term used to describe it being eaten off a naked body)

A touch of the dramatic

It's time to indulge those dress-up urges for role-play night. Doctors and nurses, strangers in a bar, boss and employee, fitness instructor and gym goer . . . whatever your fantasy, this is your moment to live it out together. Use whatever costumes and props you need to help you set the scene. Playing a character can help you to lose inhibitions and your usual patterns, which can only be a good thing for your bedroom antics.

Get your groove on

There is something about getting up close and personal with your partner on the dance floor that can really make sparks fly. Why not try something new together by signing up to a sexy dance class? It doesn't really matter whether you are any good at it or not; what makes it fun is moving together in ways you haven't tried before and using body language to communicate. Here are some ideas to light up the dance floor:

 Bachata—salsa's sensual cousin comes with close contact and lots of hip movement

♥ Rumba—the ultimate game of seduction

♥ Burlesque—learn a routine to impress your partner in the bedroom

Anyone for a dip?

We're not talking about the type you dunk
your tortilla chips in. Surprise your sweetheart
with an invitation to take a late-night visit to
a secluded spot at the beach or a lake and go
for a skinny dip together. Peeling off your layers
of clothes in front of each other is half the fun.
But the real thrill comes in diving in
the cold night water and holding each
other as the goose bumps set in. When it's
time to get out, head straight for a cozy
blanket where you can get warm together . . .
and maybe a little steamy.

Dirty
CONVERSATION
STARTERS

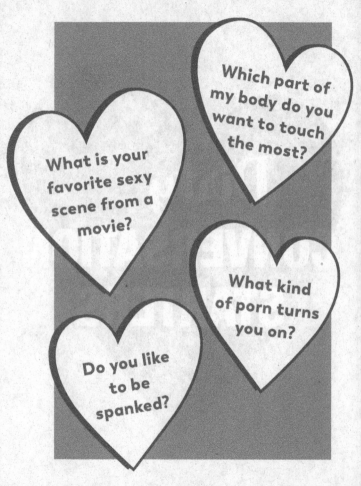

Which part of my body do you want to touch the most?

What is your favorite sexy scene from a movie?

What kind of porn turns you on?

Do you like to be spanked?

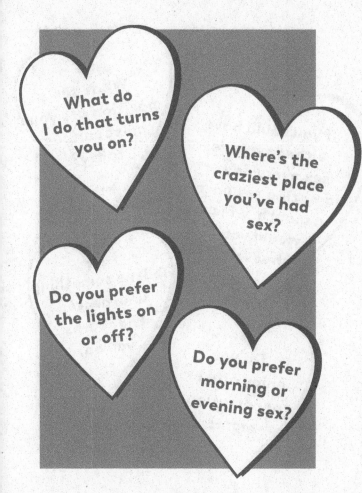

What do I do that turns you on?

Where's the craziest place you've had sex?

Do you prefer the lights on or off?

Do you prefer morning or evening sex?

21

What sex position are you most curious to try?

If you could have either average sex every day or amazing sex once a month, which would you choose?

Tell me something unexpected that turns you on.

Do you enjoy oral or penetration more?

22

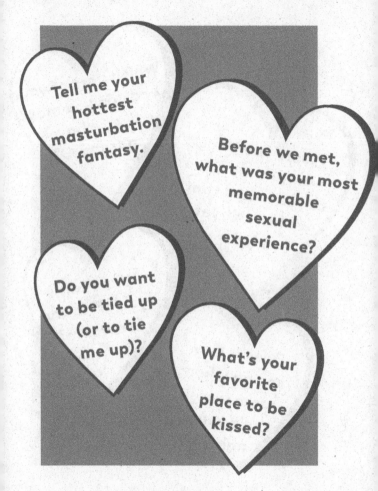

Tell me your hottest masturbation fantasy.

Before we met, what was your most memorable sexual experience?

Do you want to be tied up (or to tie me up)?

What's your favorite place to be kissed?

23

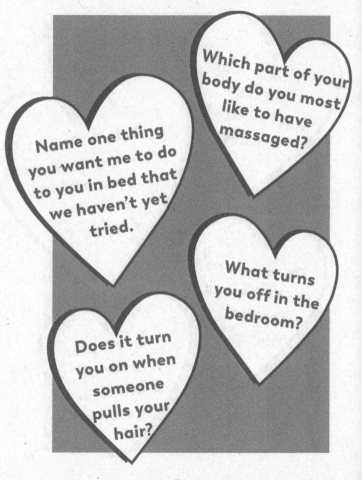

Which part of your body do you most like to have massaged?

Name one thing you want me to do to you in bed that we haven't yet tried.

What turns you off in the bedroom?

Does it turn you on when someone pulls your hair?

What's the longest you've gone without having sex?

Name a steamy vacation location where you would like to do it.

What is the weirdest sex dream you've had about a partner?

Which color underwear do you most like me to wear?

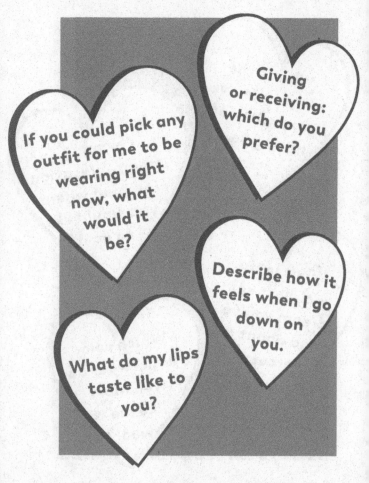

If you could pick any outfit for me to be wearing right now, what would it be?

Giving or receiving: which do you prefer?

Describe how it feels when I go down on you.

What do my lips taste like to you?

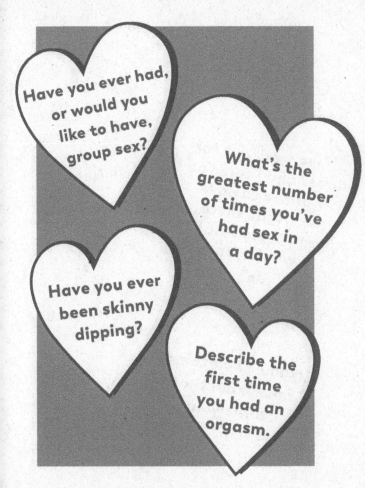

Have you ever had, or would you like to have, group sex?

What's the greatest number of times you've had sex in a day?

Have you ever been skinny dipping?

Describe the first time you had an orgasm.

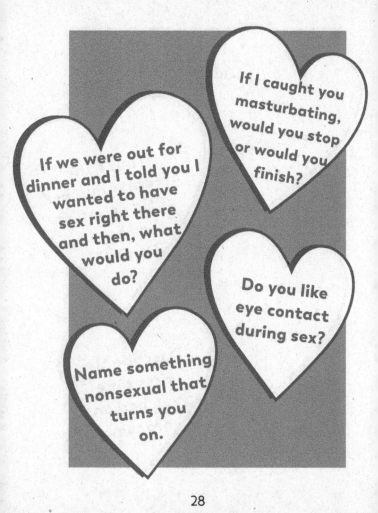

If I caught you masturbating, would you stop or would you finish?

If we were out for dinner and I told you I wanted to have sex right there and then, what would you do?

Do you like eye contact during sex?

Name something nonsexual that turns you on.

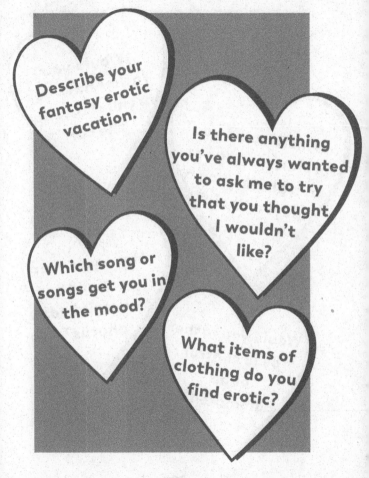

Describe your fantasy erotic vacation.

Is there anything you've always wanted to ask me to try that you thought I wouldn't like?

Which song or songs get you in the mood?

What items of clothing do you find erotic?

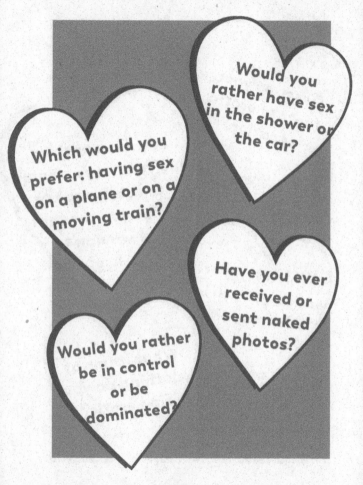

Would you rather have sex in the shower or the car?

Which would you prefer: having sex on a plane or on a moving train?

Have you ever received or sent naked photos?

Would you rather be in control or be dominated?

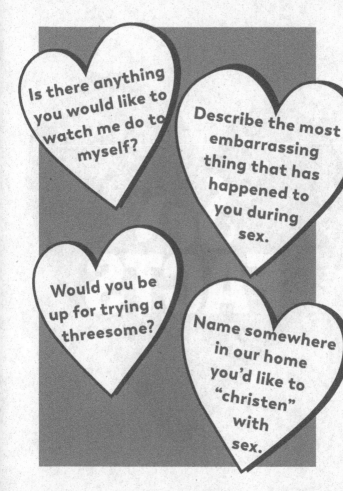

Is there anything you would like to watch me do to myself?

Describe the most embarrassing thing that has happened to you during sex.

Would you be up for trying a threesome?

Name somewhere in our home you'd like to "christen" with sex.

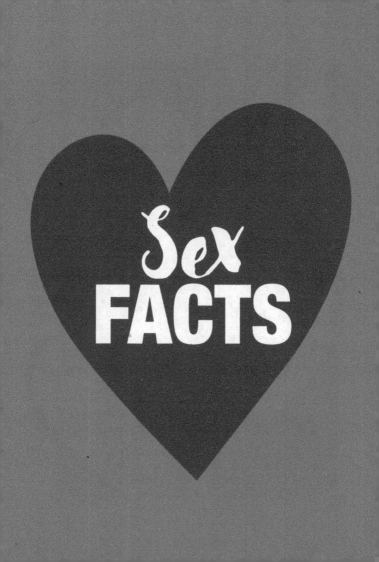

In bed with a sore head

"Not tonight, darling. I have a headache." That old excuse could be on its way out, thanks to a study conducted at the Wake Forest University School of Medicine in North Carolina, USA. The researchers discovered that migraine sufferers reported higher levels of sexual desire.

You can leave your socks on

According to researchers at the University of Groningen in the Netherlands, keeping your socks on during sex will increase your chance of having an orgasm. The theory goes that you need to be totally relaxed to orgasm, and having cold feet can hamper this. Whether you go for cute fluffy socks or sexy stockings is up to you!

No semen doesn't mean no orgasm

Did you know that, for men, an orgasm and ejaculation are two separate things? Rather than happening at the same time, the orgasm occurs slightly before ejaculation and tapers off during ejaculation. Men can learn to distinguish between the two and practice "semen retention."

Sweet wet dreams

A study published by the American Academy of Sleep Medicine found that almost one in ten of our dreams feature sex on some level. While women were more likely to have naughty dreams about their exes, celebrities or politicians, men tended to dream about having sex with more than one partner at once.

* ⭐ *

Post-coital weepies are a thing

Ever had a little cry after sex? You're not alone. There's even a name for it: post-coital dysphoria (PCD). Little is known about the condition, but certified sex therapist Ian Kerner believes that the surge in hormones after orgasm can trigger feelings of sadness, anger and even distress. So be sure to keep tissues by the bed.

* ⭐ *

The best anti-aging treatment

Having sex several times a week can keep you looking 7–12 years younger, researchers at the Royal Edinburgh Hospital in Scotland found. Regular romps release hormones, including testosterone and oestrogen, which help keep the body looking full of health and life.

Women can get it up

Although a female's genitals are smaller than a male's, they can still get an erection. The clitoris is made up of a type of spongy erectile tissue that expands with blood during arousal—just like the penis.

The better your sense of smell, the better your orgasm

According to a study published in the *Archives of Sexual Behavior*, women with a better sense of smell reported having better orgasms—and this wasn't linked to sexual desire or performance. The researchers suggested that the heightened state of pleasure experienced by these women was due to them being more readily able to detect body odors from vaginal fluid and sweat.

Sex is good for creativity

When you have sex with your partner, it releases oxytocin, which helps you to feel closer to them. But this powerful hormone also has another effect: it can create flexible cognitive pathways in the brain, which play an important role in creative thinking and can improve problem-solving.

Sex on the brain

According to Justin Lehmiller, a research fellow
at the Kinsey Institute in the US and author of a study
on sexual fantasies, 97% of us fantasize between
several times per week and several times per day.

There isn't a G-spot

The term "G-spot" is something of a misnomer.
There is an area of the urethral sponge that is very sensitive
for most people. However, researchers have not been able to
pinpoint a specific erogenous zone. So even though you may
identify your "G-spot," it won't be the same for everyone.

A natural painkiller

When we are aroused and orgasm, oxytocin is released
by the hypothalamus in the brain. According to researchers
at Rutgers University in New Jersey, USA, it is this surge
in oxytocin that can help reduce pain felt in women,
particularly during menstruation.

It's bigger than you think it is

The clitoris, that tiny love bud that brings so much pleasure, is just the tip of the iceberg. Underneath the skin lies a much larger part, the clitourethrovaginal complex, which also engorges with arousal.

Do it for the sperm

A study by the European Society of Human Reproduction and Embryology has found that having frequent sex can improve a man's sperm quality and increase fertility. The researchers found that the sperm of men who had sex or ejaculated daily was more viable and of higher quality after seven days, compared to the sperm of men who did not have sex.

Fancy condoms aren't all that

Condoms that are ribbed, or have bumps, ridges and ticklers, don't do anything to improve pleasure for the woman. The vagina is fairly insensitive to pain and stimulation—there are even some surgeries that can be performed on the vagina without the need for anaesthetics. So, it turns out the slogan "ribbed for her pleasure" was a bit of a con.

Sex is good for your career

Researchers at Oregon State University have
discovered a link between having a fulfilling sex life
and feeling more satisfied and engaged in the workplace.
So if you're going for a promotion, it might help to have
more sex with your partner (and not with your boss).

The secret to sleep success

If you're having trouble dropping off, a round of
bedroom fun might be just what you need.
After orgasm, there is a drop in dopamine and a rise
in prolactin, which has a calming effect and brings feelings
of satisfaction and sleepiness, particularly for men.

Use it or lose it

When the clitoris doesn't receive enough blood flow,
a medical condition known as clitoral atrophy can occur.
It causes the clitoris to retract into the body and a loss of
sexual sensation. Atrophy of the penis can also happen;
however, it's more often caused by injury
or ageing than lack of sex.

Wear flats for the win

Did you know that the arch in the high-heeled shoes
produced by certain high-end shoe brands is intended to
recreate the arch in a woman's pelvis during orgasm?
Unfortunately, because walking around in the heels from
day to day creates a contraction in the pelvic floor,
it cannot contract further during orgasm,
leading to a less satisfying experience.

Bless you!

During sex, the genitals and breasts swell, but did you know
that in some people, the inner nose can swell too? This causes
congestion, sometimes known as "honeymoon nose." It is due
to the presence of erectile tissue in the nose, which becomes
engorged during arousal. There is also a related condition in
which people sneeze uncontrollably during sex.

Love at first scent

The writers of a paper published in *Frontiers in Psychology*
found that smell plays an important role in attraction.
While odors that were identified as more pleasant
and sexier made people want to flirt or date, unpleasant odors
were found to have the opposite effect.

Take a seat—but not for too long

Sitting in a chair can sometimes lead to a woman feeling aroused. That's because it presses on the pudendal nerves, underneath the buttocks and the sitting bones, which feed arousal tissues in the vagina, clitoris and anus. However, sitting in a chair all day can also have a negative effect on sexual pleasure, because it shortens the pelvic floor and psoas muscles. These muscles become tight from sitting too much, making it harder for women to achieve a good orgasm.

No two vaginas are the same

Just as the pattern of a snowflake is unique, the nerve endings in the vagina are distributed differently in every woman. That's why slightly different methods are needed to achieve orgasm for every individual.

Pardon me?

The German word for contraceptive is *Schwangerschaftsverhütungsmittel* (literally: pregnancy prevention medicine.) By the time you've got that tongue twister out, it's probably too late!

Nature's love potion

During the 12-to-48-hour window when a fertile woman is ovulating (and can get pregnant), typical alpha males will find her more attractive than when she's not ovulating. In a study in which men rated the armpit odors of women at various stages in their menstrual cycle, participants marked the smells that came from women who were ovulating as most attractive. Another study discovered that men find the *faces* of ovulating women more attractive.

✦ ✦ ✦

Too much going solo is a no-no

"Delayed ejaculation" is the term used for men who find it difficult to orgasm in conventional ways. According to clinical sexologist Cyndi Darnell, one reason this can happen is if a man develops an "idiosyncratic masturbation style," meaning that they become so used to a specific combination of pressure and speed from masturbating that they find it difficult to replicate that with a partner, whether through penetration or oral sex.

Ginger gets you going

Ginger has many health benefits, including reducing nausea and soothing sore throats. But did you know that it could also amp up sexual excitement? Research has suggested that it could increase blood flow, reduce oxidative stress and enhance fertility in men and women. So, it's likely to help you get geared up for bedroom antics. Ginger tea, anyone?

* * *

Maneuver with care

Ever heard of a penile fracture? Unfortunately, it is a real thing, though thankfully it is rare. It is most likely to occur when a couple switches position while the erect penis is in the vagina, though it can also happen during over-enthusiastic thrusting. So take it easy there, cowboy!

* * *

You need those Zs

A study by psychologists at Hendrix College in Arkansas, USA, revealed that sleep deprivation in men could result in them incorrectly perceiving that women are interested in having sex with them. The moral of the story?
Before you make a move, sleep on it.

Bedroom workout

The official figures are in: a study at the University of
Montreal in Canada concluded that having sex burns
an average of 100 calories for men. The number of
calories burned by women is ... 69.

Off to a stiff start

Morning glory, morning wood, slumber lumber ...
The official medical term for getting an erection while
still snoozing in the morning is nocturnal penile
tumescence. Remember that the next time you're
teased for sporting a breakfast boner.

Wake up and smell the pumpkins

The Smell and Taste Treatment and Research
Foundation in Chicago, USA, conducted a study into
which smells turn a man on. They discovered that the
odor of pumpkin significantly increased blood flow to
the penis. The effect was even more powerful when
pumpkin was mixed with lavender, and, to a lesser
extent, when combined with doughnuts.

Keep your cholesterol in check

High cholesterol is bad for the body in many ways, but did you know that it can also impair sexual function? In fact, it can even lead to erectile dysfunction. Researchers at Rutgers University's Robert Wood Johnson Medical School in the US found that, when people took cholesterol-lowering medication, they were eventually able to enjoy better sex.

* * *

Sex sells

It's not just the modern generation that is obsessed with sex. In the fifteenth century, the best-selling work of fiction was an erotic novel called *The Tale of the Two Lovers*, written, rather surprisingly, by the man who later became Pope Pius II.

* * *

A sporting chance

In 2012, the Olympics were held in London, UK, and lasted 17 days. Among the items provided for the visiting athletes were 150,000 free condoms—which works out to about 15 per person. It's not known whether the athletes managed to get through all the condoms, but if they did, after their physically demanding days in the arena, that's impressive!

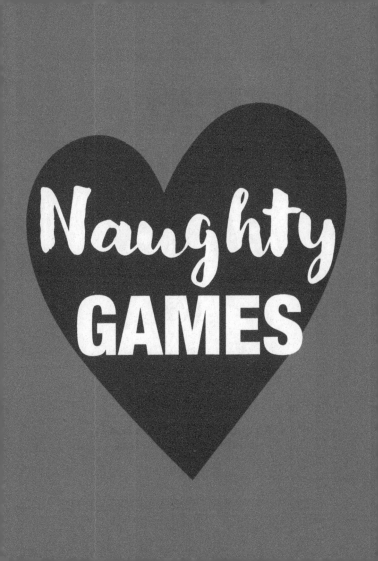

TICKLE YOUR FANCY

You will need:

A feather

A blindfold

An outline of a human body
(naughty bits included)

A pen

How to Play

Prepare for some ticklish fun by printing out an outline of a human body. Or, you could tape together a few sheets of newspaper and draw around your partner for a life-sized version. Pin your outline to the wall and blindfold your partner.

Turn them around a few times and guide them to the poster. They must mark three places to tickle you, using the pen. It's up to you how much you help them, but bear in mind that any marks that don't land on the outline won't count for the next stage of the game. Maybe you'll surprise them by guiding them to a sensitive spot they don't know about.

Take the blindfold off: it's time to be tickled! There's no time limit for this part of the game. If they've picked a certain area that really turns you on, tell them to keep going and even ask them to nibble or suck that spot instead.

When you can't take any more, swap roles and don the blindfold.

SPIN THE DILDO

You will need:

A dildo

A silk scarf

A spanking tool

A jar of honey

An egg timer

How to Play

Set out the silk scarf, spanking tool and jar of honey in a circle, with the dildo in the center. (If you don't have a dildo, you can of course use a bottle.)

Take it in turns to spin the dildo. If the knob-end comes to a stop pointing at empty space, then your partner is "safe" for this turn and it passes to them.

If the knob-end points at the silk scarf, you can either blindfold your partner or tie their hands together with the scarf. Start the egg timer (or set a time limit on your phone) and do what you will with them until the buzzer goes off.

If the knob-end points at the spanking tool, give your partner a spanking—or ask for one yourself, whichever gives you the most pleasure.

If the knob-end points at the jar of honey, dab a bit of honey on the part of your body that you want your partner to lick or suck.

SEXY SIX

You will need:

Two dirty minds

How to Play

Think of something that really turns you on. It could be your favorite sex position, a particularthingyourpartnerdoestoyouorthe part of your body you most love them to kiss or touch.

Your partner now gets to ask you six questions, to which you can only answer "yes" or "no," to try to work out what you're thinking.

If they guess correctly, then the turn passes to them.

If they guess incorrectly, they have to act out what you were thinking about.

REMEMBER WHEN . . .

You will need:

A set of handcuffs

A blindfold

How to Play

The active player should be fully dressed but with sexy underwear underneath. The passive player should be wearing just their underwear.

Handcuff your partner to a chair or bed, then kick things off by asking them, "Remember when . . . ?" and giving them a prompt to recall a saucy moment in your relationship. For every detail they remember correctly, remove one item of your clothing. If they answer incorrectly, blindfold them. The game continues until you are down to your sexy smalls . . . or you get distracted.

NAUGHTY
NUMBERS

You will need:

A pack of cards

Sparkling wine

How to Play

Shuffle the deck and place it face down between you. Cut the cards to see who goes first (ace is low). The player who won the cut turns over the top card. The cards relate to actions that the players must do, as follows:

♥ **Ace, 2 or 3:** the other player takes off an item of their clothing.

♥ **4, 5 or 6:** the card turner takes off an item of their clothing.

♥ **7, 8 or 9:** the other player pours sparkling wine down themselves and the card turner licks it off.

♥ **10:** the card turner gets a promise from the other player of something naughty that you will do together later.

♥ **Jack, queen and king:** play passes to the other player.

Continue until either or both of you are completely naked or the sparkling wine is finished, whichever (or whoever) comes first.

WET
T-SHIRT
FUN

You will need:

Water guns

Buckets

Balloons

White T-shirts

Plenty of water

How to Play

Strip down to just your underwear, don the white T-shirts and head to a spot suitable for nudity and water sports—so an oversized bathroom or a back garden that's not overlooked.

Prepare your selection of watery missiles: fill up the water guns, bombs and buckets.

Take turns asking each other questions to test your knowledge of each other's sexual likes and dislikes. For example:

💜 What's my favorite place to be licked?

💜 What's the best time we've ever had sex?

💜 In what public place would I like to do it?

For every question your partner gets wrong, give them a good dousing.

Keep going till your underwear and T-shirts leave nothing to the imagination.

SEXY
SLEUTHING

You will need:

Your own clothes

Some sexy underwear

Candles

Rose petals

Sticky notes

A pen

How to Play

In this game, your partner will need to use their sleuthing skills to track down a saucy reward: you! You will need to do some preparation before your partner arrives home and send them a notification when the game is afoot.

Hide the clothes you've been wearing in different spots around the house.

On sticky notes, write clues that will lead your partner from one clothes item to the next, working their way from your coat down to your underwear, which should have the final clue attached to it—the one that will lead them to you.

In your chosen spot, lie naked, surrounded by rose petals and candles, ready for them to enjoy their reward.

ROLL FOR LICKS

You will need:

A few bars of chocolate

A die

How to Play

Melt the chocolate in a big bowl and place it in the middle of the room.

Sit on either side of the bowl and each take a roll of the die. Whoever rolls the highest gets to smear chocolate over a body part of the other player.

Repeat until you both have a generous coating of chocolate.

The play now goes up a gear: whoever rolls highest gets to select which of their body parts the other player should lick clean.

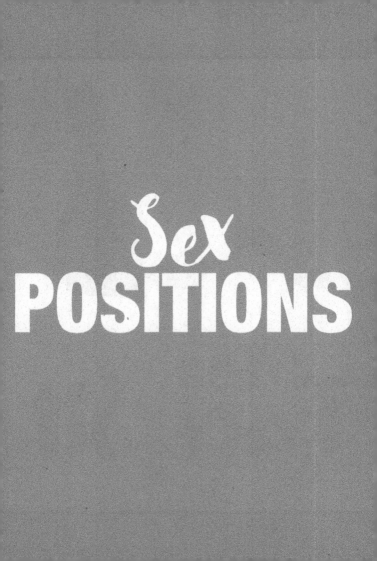

Sex
POSITIONS

The
Face Sit

There's nothing like a tickle on the inner thigh to get the party started, and this position will provide ample opportunity for just that. This oral classic is perfect for those who like to tease and those who like to be teased.

The giver lies down on their back, while the receiver kneels over the giver's face, lowering their body until their naughty parts are in reach of the giver's tongue. The receiver is in control here, and they can tease the giver by moving away just out of reach.

The receiver can hold on to the wall or bedframe to keep themselves steady, or the giver can support the receiver by holding on to their behind, throwing in a cheeky bottom squeeze.

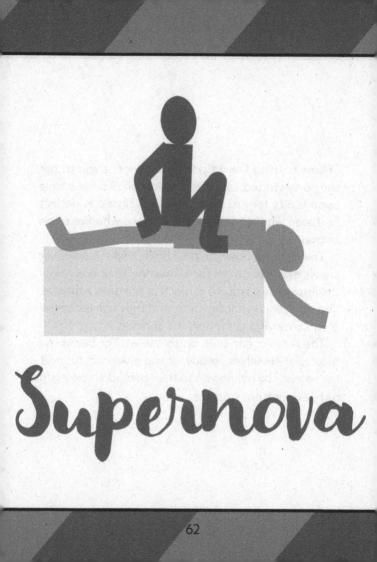

Supernova

Send your partner off on a trip to the stars with this stratospheric sexual position that will keep them hanging until the explosive end.

Proceedings start with the passive partner lying on their back on the bed, with their head near to the edge of the bed. The active partner straddles them and rocks back and forth until both partners are almost reaching *their* edge.

At this point the active partner stops, puts weight through their knees and shifts their partner towards the edge of the bed so their head, shoulders and arms hang down.

The active partner resumes rocking until they both come. The blood rushing to the passive partner's head will intensify their orgasm.

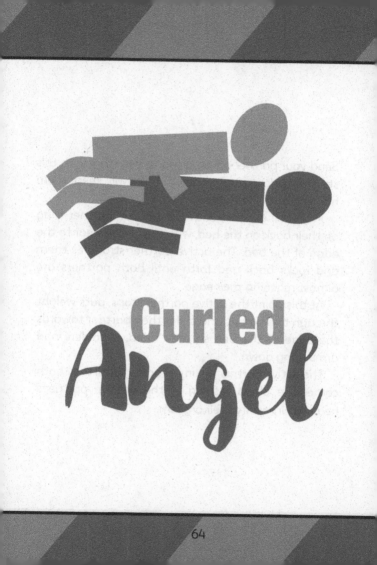

Curled
Angel

This cozy position is perfect for couples who like to spoon . . . and mix in a bit of forking.

The little spoon curls up with their partner behind them, allowing the big spoon to penetrate them with ease. They can also reach around to add to the passive partner's pleasure with their hand.

This gentle position is ideal for pregnant women because it avoids squashing the baby bump.

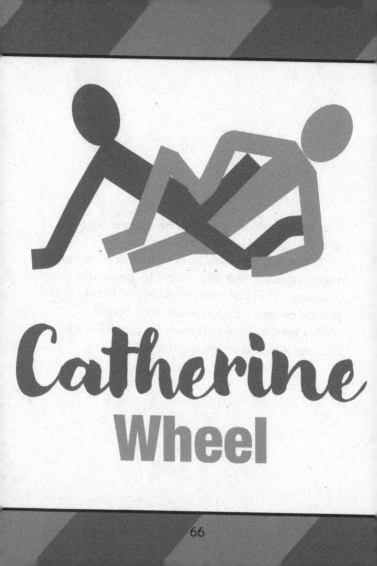

Catherine
Wheel

Take your seats for this intertwined position that gives perfect penetration or frottage results. For the uninitiated, frottage means rubbing your parts together. Be ready for fireworks!

Sit facing one another and shift towards each other until your naughty bits touch.

Wrap your legs around each other, lean back and rest your hands on the bed or floor for support.

Start with a gentle grinding motion and build in intensity until you're both ready to explode.

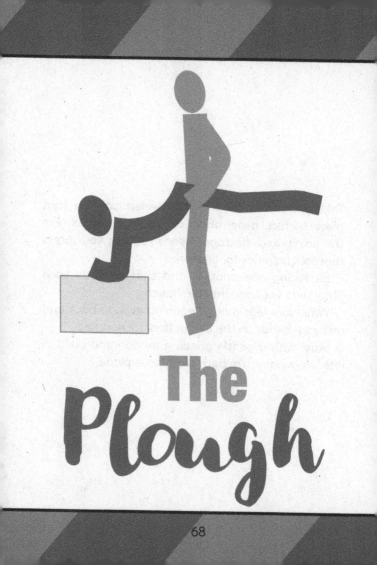

The Plough

Remember the wheelbarrow race at school sports day? Those skills are about to come in handy for this energetic position. The active partner takes full control and needs a good bit of stamina to see this through to the end.

The passive partner lies on their front at the end of the bed, legs over the edge, while the active partner lifts the passive partner's legs, holds on to their hips and moves in for penetration.

The passive partner uses their elbows for support while the active partner holds them up and takes care of business from behind.

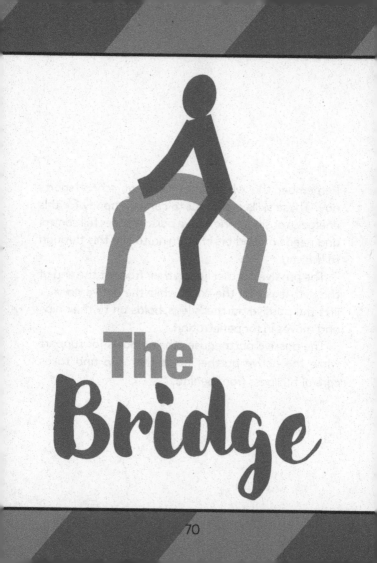

The Bridge

This advanced position is one for the yogis and definitely not for the faint-hearted. The active partner should probably practice ahead of time to make sure they've got the strength to hold the position.

The active partner bends over backwards to form a bridge, and the passive partner straddles them, lowering themselves down gently to achieve penetration.

The roles switch up here, as the passive partner becomes active, using the motion of their legs to control penetration.

You might want to ramp up the foreplay before moving into the position so that you don't have to stay in it too long. Your blood will be rushing to your head!

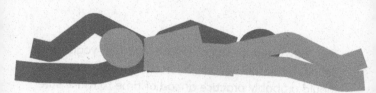

Side 69

Take it easy with this horizontal position that lets you focus your energy on pleasuring your partner. It's just like the classic 69 position, but instead of being one on top of the other, the partners lie side by side facing each other, their faces nuzzled between their partner's legs.

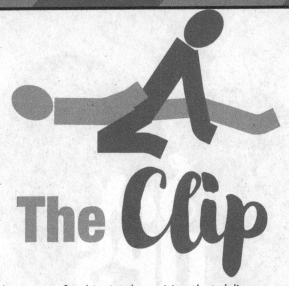

The Clip

Hop on top for this simple position that delivers every time.

The passive partner lies on their back with their legs closed. The active partner straddles them and leans back on their hands, allowing for penetration and giving their partner a great view.

The partner up top then builds rhythm using a sliding movement, perfectly positioned for the passive partner to reach out and add manual stimulation to the mix.

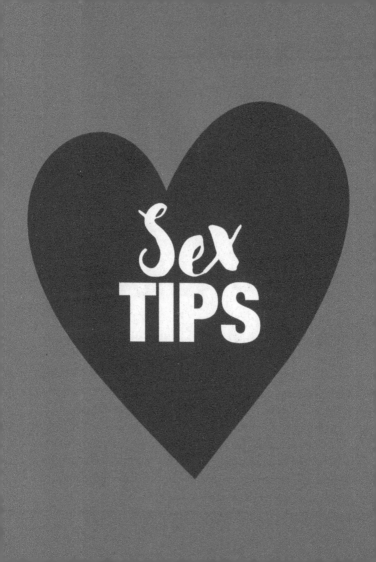

Sex
TIPS

Pre-game fun and games

They say that foreplay is the best part of sex.
Even better—you don't have to wait until you're
in the bedroom together to get it started.
Give your partner a taste of what's to come by
sending them suggestive texts throughout the
day, or whisper your sexy plans in their ear while
you're out in public. The more detailed you are,
the better, so that they have plenty of fuel for
their wicked imagination. By the time you're
finally alone together, you'll be ripping each
other's clothes off so that you can execute that
naughty playbook of moves.

Take a breather

Sometimes the beauty of a kiss lies in the pre-kiss anticipation. This tantric breathing exercise will draw out that exquisite moment until you can take it no more. (NB: A quick breath check and brush of the teeth might be a good idea before you begin.)

To really relax into the moment, lie down side by side and facing each other. With your lips parted, breathe deeply in and out in an opposing rhythm: while you breathe out, your partner breathes in, and while they breathe out, you breathe in.

An alternative option is to synchronize your breathing—in through your noses and out through your mouths—while staring into each other's eyes.

Nipple *tease*

Did you know that nipples have hundreds of nerve endings?
That makes them the perfect focus point for some foreplay
action. This two-step titillating trick
will get your partner's senses tingling in no time.

 Step one: relax your lips and swirl your
tongue around one of your partner's nipples.

 Step two: gently poke the nipple with
the tip of your tongue.

Switch back and forth between the two steps until
your partner begs for more. And when they do, tease
out the tension by withholding for as long as you can
stand it. Simple, but oh so effective.

Celebrate the past

Good memories are the foundation of a relationship. And what better way to celebrate what you have than by reliving some of your finest moments together? Take it in turns to recall an intense snapshot from your romantic timeline, whether that be your first flirtations, your first kiss, the first time you had sex—or the wildest time. The saucy devil is in the details here, so try to give as many as you can. Your reminiscing session is bound to get those nerve endings tingling. When you both agree on a favorite, it's time to stage your very own re-enactment. Who said history can't be fun?

For the very first time

There's nothing quite like the thrill of meeting someone for the first time and feeling those sparks fly. Well, actually, there is. This classic role-play gives couples all the excitement of an illicit liaison, without the cheating.

Send your partner a text arranging to meet in a bar. Use a pre-agreed code word so that they know the role-play is afoot. Arrive at the bar separately and sit apart. To get the ball rolling, one of you will have to introduce yourself to the other—just like chatting a stranger up in a bar. To get the best out of the role-play, give yourselves different names, occupations and backstories. That will give you plenty to talk about on your "first meeting." And when things progress "back to theirs/yours," that's where the real fun begins. Hey, if it works for Claire and Phil Dunphy in *Modern Family*, it can work for you.

Dirty talk
is overrated

They say that communication is key, and that's true, but it doesn't only have to be about verbal communication. Getting what you want without having to ask for it holds a special pleasure of its own. In this tip, you and your partner will focus on sensation and touch, which will help to strengthen your physical connection.

To kick things off, without saying a word, put your hands on each other's intimate parts. When your partner does something that's pleasurable for you, respond in kind by rubbing, stroking or squeezing—whatever you know they like. You'll soon start to understand why silence is golden.

Playing with the senses

When you deny a person one of their senses,
it only serves to heighten all the others.
Use this knowledge to your advantage
for a bit of bedroom fun.

Try blindfolding your partner and describe
exactly what you're going to do to them . . .
or yourself. If you're both feeling more
adventurous, handcuff your partner.
Tell them that they can look but they can't
touch while you do what you will with them.

If this isn't your thing, there are subtler ways
to engage the senses. Treat your partner to a
sensual massage using aromatherapy oils.
Patchouli, ylang-ylang and geranium are great
options, but choose whichever your partner
responds to best. Start by warming a drop of
the oil in your hands and hold it under your
partner's nose so they get the full sensory
experience of breathing in the scent.

The long way up

Giving your partner a back massage is a great way to get them feeling relaxed, but in this massage, you'll also be amping up the sexual tension.

Invite your partner to get comfortable on the bed, but instead of lying face down, suggest that they lie face up. You could add a drop of sensual essential oil to a blindfold and drape it over their eyes.

Begin at the bottom and slowly work your way up, starting with their feet, moving up to their calves, pausing to give a bit of teasing attention behind the knee, then moving on to the inner thighs. By the time you reach their groin, they'll be quivering with anticipation. Of course, it's up to you whether you finish with a happy ending.

You don't have to take your clothes off

Stripping off for your partner is hot, but how about when you want each other so bad you haven't got time to get properly undressed? That can be even hotter. Switch things up a gear by telling your partner you must have them right away. Underwear pulled to the side (or even better, surprise your partner by not wearing any underwear), skirt pushed up, shirt buttons flying off . . . do whatever you need to do to get to each other in the heat of the moment.

Or why not take a trip back to those teenage days of illicit fun by not getting undressed at all? Having "outercourse" can be a way to spice things up if they've got a little repetitive in the bedroom. Just whisper "Let's pretend we're not allowed to have sex" in your partner's ear, and it's a dry hump to the finish line.

Taking things to the extreme

Very hot and very cold temperatures can set your senses alight and send shivers down your spine, especially when they are introduced during the throes of passion. This is because the change in temperature stimulates sensory glands, not to mention the titillating "pleasure and pain" combination that it brings to the table. Here are a few ideas to set your senses tingling:

♥ Drip warm oil or wax on your partner

♥ Pleasure your partner with a pre-chilled sex toy

♥ Rub an ice cube around their nipple

♥ Touch your partner in a private sauna

Come and watch the show

The list of positive side effects of masturbation is long. Scientists all seem to agree that knocking one off is a healthy way of getting a mood-boosting endorphin hit. But it's even more fun when you have a masturbation buddy. Create a little bespoke porn show for yourselves by watching each other get off. If you've never tried masturbating in front of someone else before, ease yourself into it by touching yourself everywhere but your genitals first. Part of the fun is watching your partner watching you, and watching them back. When you can't control yourself any longer, look each other in the eyes as you both head for the finish line.

All the angles

Have you ever wanted to know what you and your partner look like having sex? Of course, you could record your very own sex tape together, but if the thought of seeing yourself on screen makes you cringe, or you don't have the right technological setup, a bit of mirror-facing action can be just as fun (and it's probably safer in the long run.) Position a full-length mirror opposite your bed and off you go. You can use your reflection for some mind-blowing eye contact or check out the full view while you bone.

Bare-naked ambition

Save yourselves a trip to the beauty salon by treating each other to an at-home pubic grooming session. Start with a hot bath so your skin and pubic hair are soft. If shaving is your thing, let your partner foam you up and shave you down with a razor. If you prefer wax, mix pleasure with pain as your partner applies hot wax to you and pulls it off (be sure to follow the package instructions carefully to avoid injury, of course!). When you're both nice and smooth, why not finish with a lazy Side 69 (see page 72)?

Phone fun

Picture the scene: your partner's away
on a work trip, or you're stuck housesitting
for your aunt. Night has fallen, and you've
got the raging horn. If only your lover was there.
Sigh. Well, guess what? The sexy
fun doesn't have to stop just because
you're separated. Thanks to modern
technology, sizzling phone sex is only
ever a click away. To add some extra fun
to your remote love session, why not invest
in some remote-controlled sex toys that
can be controlled using smartphone apps? And
if your partner's ever not available,
you also have the option of some solo fun.

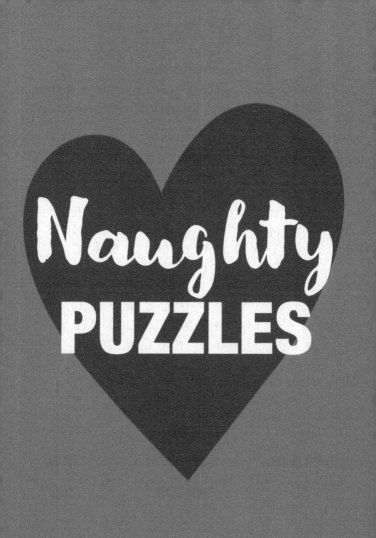

WORDSEARCH

Touch me there

Find nine places to touch or kiss your partner that
will drive them wild, hidden in the wordsearch.

```
U K W J O B T S U A J N P A T
S P C E M I U K A P G Q W V G
H H L A A P M Z R S R V K W A
J A O F B N M N M S C H G N H
X J B U V R Y U P E W I U F G
T X M F L M E F I Y H G W N U
Y P I W O D B W T U T S L C L
K V Q K Z U E D O W U O S R Y
P X G A T R T R R L O U M L X
R U C T N I P P L E M V L Q I
V Y O K B M C W E B Q Q K J B
B C C T B B Y H A L W Q N X Y
K E Y H K Z R Z O O F A Y G I
N L B V L L R B Q I S R R N V
Z S X R A E F Q W E F U Z N X
```

ARMPIT	BUTTOCK	EAR
LOWER BACK	MOUTH	NECK
NIPPLE	SHOULDER	TUMMY

WORD
Ladder

Change GIVE into HEAD by altering one letter at a time to make a new word on each step of the ladder.

G I V E

_ _ _ _

_ _ _ _

_ _ _ _

H E A D

ANAGRAMS

Rearrange the letters to reveal the titles of some naughty movies.

EARTHED POT
TELEVISED JOHNS MINIS
HORNED GOLFS

CROSSWORD

Sex on the brain
Solve the naughty-themed clues
to complete this crossword.

ACROSS

2. Assume this position for a wild ride

3. Meg Ryan had a fake one at a
   diner in *When Harry Met Sally*

4. Lover of feet

5. One who hasn't had sex yet

DOWN

1. Sexual literature or art

2. Fictional writer of New York sex column

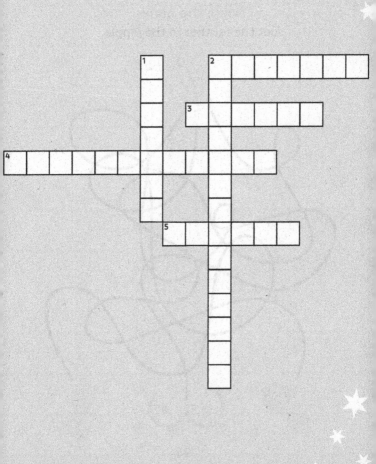

MAZE

Tickle the nipple

Get the feather to the nipple.

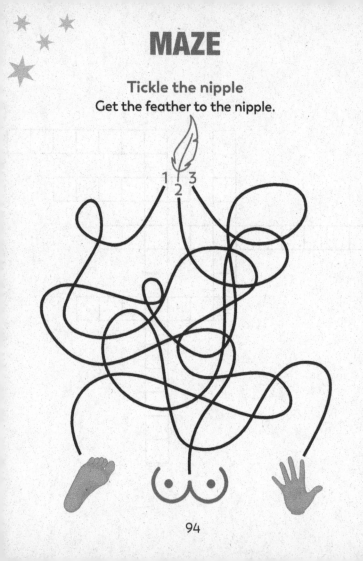

WORDSEARCH

Sexy accessories

Find nine bedside cabinet essentials
hidden in the wordsearch.

```
X D I N E X H Y P L Z R W L B
A J N C G G D C K Q O W G I L
D J N S E U S S I T W U N O I
E V R I O D Z D A Z L R L E N
H S F C P B Y R D P K L E G D
S L O S F P B F L V X E J A F
C M U K L I L A X R T G Q S F
L L O U V E N E K E A O A S L
P V B D H A N D C U F F S A D
W E Y W N K E I Z L U Y G M F
P H M C I O J F H F A W P K H
Z U W G B K C M Z I W M P G F
F E F R S L I Y A J S J P M D
E K K Z I G C Z O V L I T S V
H W X H Z V W P A Z L O P M O
```

ANAL PLUG   BLINDFOLD   CONDOMS

HANDCUFFS   LUBE   MASSAGE OIL

NIPPLE CLAMPS   TISSUES   VIBRATOR

WORD
Ladder

Change PULL into SUCK by altering one letter at a time to make a new word on each step of the ladder.

P U L L

_ _ _ _

_ _ _ _

_ _ _ _

S U C K

ANAGRAMS

Rearrange the letters to reveal the titles of three sexual pursuits.

SLUICING NUN
LEAF TOIL
INNATE TROPE

MAZE

Lick the lolly
Get the tongue to the lolly.

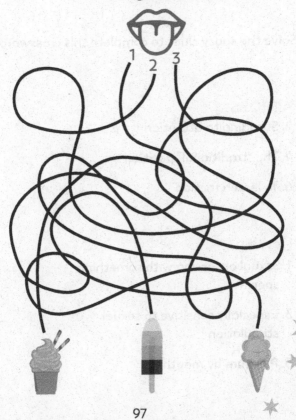

CROSSWORD

All about sex
Solve the saucy clues to complete this crossword.

ACROSS

2. Standing to attention

4. The "traditional" position

6. To lessen friction

DOWN

1. Sexual obsession with something specific

3. Especially sensitive to sexual stimulation

5. Pleasure by mouth

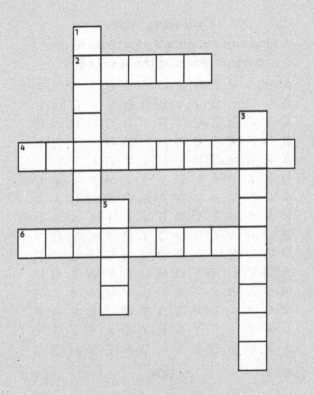

WORDSEARCH

Titillating tricks

Find nine naughty things to do to your
partner hidden in the wordsearch.

```
S B B V Z N J O G S U S T T E
A U O L B J V U R D K I Q Q L
K Y C A Z C D P B H C U H W D
X O F K T B B H H K H Y I Z L
K R A M E D L H L Z Q C B N I
N X K I A L D E J F M Y L V L
I G S V S V B R H F H H D F P
K C I L E L F B V K I K I B P
B U P W K B Q O I Q Y N Y U Y
O W U S A P R O K N G Z C R F
D Q Z L R P U N U E F W C F M
M J I W J P A Y R V V W Y T Z
V G Y K P P Q S T R O K E H F
L A B J S T G R K O K E L Z Y
F X D D G K T K O M E V H O G
```

FINGER	LICK	NIBBLE
RUB	SPANK	STROKE
SUCK	TEASE	TICKLE

WORD
Ladder

Change MOAN into COME by altering one letter at a time to make a new word on each step of the ladder.

M O A N

_ _ _ _

_ _ _ _

C O M E

ANAGRAMS

Rearrange the letters to reveal three popular sex positions.

THESE TINY NIX
ROSY SIMIAN
EDGY GOT SLY

Date Night
VOUCHERS

To . . . .

I PROMISE...
...to take you
out dancing.

Signed. . . . .

Date. . . . .

To . . . .

I PROMISE...
...to write you a love poem and read it to you.

Signed. . . . .

Date. . . . .

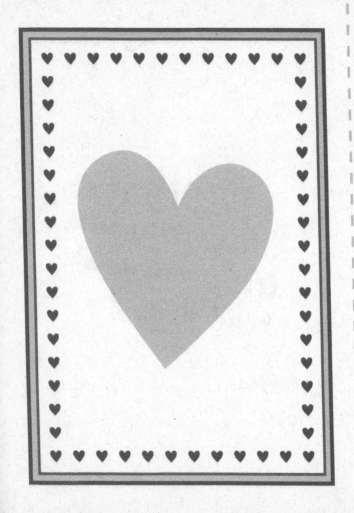

To . . . .

I PROMISE....

...to have a luxurious bath ready for you when you come home from work.

Signed . . . .

Date . . . .

To . . . .

I PROMISE...
...to take you
to see your
favorite show.

Signed. . . . .

Date. . . . .

To ....

I PROMISE....
...to surprise you
with a romantic
getaway.

Signed........................

Date........................

To ....

I PROMISE...
...to have a
lie-in with you
every Sunday
for a month.

Signed..........................

Date..........................

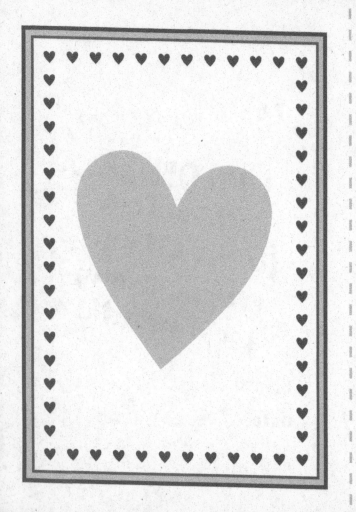

Raunchy
RECIPES

Caviar Caresses

Serves 2

These luscious mouthfuls are sure to get your senses tingling as the tiny eggs burst, oozing their slightly sweet, rich flavor over your tongue. You'll be licking your lips and ready for more.

Ingredients

- 150 ml (½ cup) sour cream
- 1 tbsp fresh chives, chopped
- 1 tbsp fresh dill, chopped (or 1 tsp dried dill)
- Black pepper, to season
- 1 cucumber
- 50 g (2 oz) caviar (such as red salmon caviar)
- Fresh dill sprigs, to garnish (optional)

Method

1. Stir the sour cream, chives, dill and a twist of black pepper together in a bowl.

2. Wash and peel the cucumber, then slice it into ½-cm (¼-inch) rounds.

3. Spread a teaspoon of the sour cream mixture on each cucumber round and top with a tiny spoonful of caviar.

4. Top with sprigs of fresh dill and enjoy.

Oysters in the Buff

Serves 2

It is often said that this shellfish resembles a most alluring part of the female anatomy. Whatever your sexual persuasion, it will be hard to hold back when faced with a platter of these moist morsels. Splash out on the highest-grade specimens as they will require very little dressing to hit the pleasure spot.

Ingredients

- 12 fresh oysters
- 24 ice cubes
- 2 lemons, cut into wedges
- Freshly ground black and white pepper
- Hot sauce

Method

1. You will want to eat these beauties raw for maximum effect, so make sure you buy from a reputable market, keep them chilled and consume on the day of purchase.

2. Give the oysters a good scrubbing to remove any grit.

3. Open them just before serving. To do so, wrap a dishtowel around one hand and hold the oyster firmly in it, with the flat side on top and the hinge towards you. Insert the sharp edge of a broad, heavy knife into the crack between the shells as close to the hinge as you can. Twist the knife until the gap pops open, then work the knife around until the halves separate easily.

4. Discard the flat side of the shells, leaving the oysters in the saucer-shaped shells. Remove any small pieces of grit or shell and loosen the oyster with a small, sharp knife.

5. Serve the oysters on a platter of ice cubes, with the lemon wedges, pepper and hot sauce on the side, to be added as taste requires.

6. Tilt your heads back, slurp and enjoy.

Balls of Fun

Serves 2

There's nothing quite like popping a juicy ball in your mouth and giving it a good suck. It's time to get some nuts with these delicious meat-free spherical snacks.

Ingredients

- 2 tbsp ground almonds
- 2 tbsp ground hazelnuts
- 2 tbsp ground pecans
- 4 tbsp fresh white breadcrumbs
- 100 g (4 oz) Cheddar cheese, grated
- 1 large egg
- 4 tbsp sherry (dry is best)—and have the bottle handy
- 1 small onion, finely sliced
- 1 red bell pepper, deseeded and sliced

into tiny chunks
- 6-cm piece fresh ginger, peeled and grated
- 1 tbsp fresh parsley, chopped
- 1 small red chilli, deseeded and finely chopped
- Salt and black pepper, to season
- 1 lemon, quartered to serve

Method

1. Stir the nuts, breadcrumbs and cheese together in a big bowl.

2. In a separate bowl, lightly beat together the egg and sherry. Mix in the onion, ginger, parsley, chilli and the red bell pepper.

3. Add the eggy mixture to the nut and cheese mix, season well with salt and pepper and knead it all together.

4. Form ten little balls half the size of your fists. If the mixture is too dry and the balls fall apart, add sherry little by little until it comes together.

5. Place the balls on a greased baking tray in the oven and turn it on (they need to heat up slowly rather than roast). Keep the heat low (180°C/350°F) and cook for 25 minutes.

6. Serve with a wedge of lemon and a sauce of your choice.

Glistening Glazed Breasts

Serves 2

Picture the plate: two perfectly formed breasts, slick with a strawberry sheen and just waiting for you to wrap your lips around them. Pink perfection!

Ingredients

- 225 g (8 oz) strawberries
- Juice and zest of 1 lemon
- 2 tbsp white wine vinegar
- 1 tbsp fresh mint, finely chopped (or 1 tsp prepared mint sauce)
- Black pepper, to season
- 2 large spring onions, finely chopped
- 2 tbsp olive oil
- 2 large chicken breasts

Method

1. Put aside a couple of strawberries to use as garnish, and blitz the rest for about a minute in a food processor.

2. Place the puréed strawberries, lemon juice and zest, vinegar, mint, a twist of pepper and onions in a bowl and mix together. Whisk the olive oil in with a fork.

3. Lay the chicken breasts in a baking tray and heap the mixture over the top. Marinate in the fridge for a few hours before cooking.

4. Heat the oven to 200°C (400°F) and place the baking tray in the center of the oven for 12–15 minutes. Baste with the strawberry mixture every 4 minutes.

5. Check the meat with a sharp knife to see if the juices run clear. Crisp the glaze a little by placing the breasts under a hot grill (broiler) for about a minute.

6. Top each breast with a strawberry.

7. Serve with rice and your best seductive smile.

Sensual Scramble

Serves 2

The heady truffle flavor of these delectable eggs will set your taste buds tingling and leave you sighing with pleasure.

Ingredients

- 4 medium eggs
- 50 g (2 oz) dark or white truffles, sliced
- 1 tbsp crème fraîche
- Salt and black pepper, to season
- Sliced bread, for toasting

Method

1. Bring a large saucepan of water to the boil.

2. In a second, smaller saucepan or bowl, drop in the eggs and gently whisk. Season lightly with salt and pepper, and add the truffles.

3. Place the smaller saucepan or bowl over the boiling water and stir the mixture continuously until it begins to thicken—usually about 5–6 minutes.

4. Remove from heat and stir in the crème fraîche.

5. Spread thickly on toast and serve immediately.

Long, Slow, Seductive Screw

Serves 2

Sip one of these, and you'll soon be ready to loosen up and get horizontal.

Ingredients

- 25 ml (1 oz) vodka
- 25 ml (1 oz) sloe gin
- 25 ml (1 oz) Southern Comfort
- 25 ml (1 oz) Galliano
- 25 ml (1 oz) amaretto
- Orange juice

Method

1. Put the alcohol ingredients in a cocktail shaker and shake to combine.

2. Pour the mix into ice-filled tall glasses.

3. Top up with orange juice and serve.

Lusty Chocolate Lick

Serves 2

It's time to get saucy with this unctuous, decadent chocolate confection.

Ingredients

- 225 g (8 oz) high-quality dark chocolate, broken into pieces
- 2 tbsp golden syrup
- 2 tbsp espresso coffee
- 300 ml (1 cup) single cream
- 1 tbsp dark rum

Method

1. Melt the chocolate, golden syrup, coffee and cream together in a glass bowl suspended over a pan, a quarter full of gently simmering water.

2. Keep stirring until the chocolate has completely melted. It should have an even consistency and a glossy texture. Stir in the rum and remove from heat.

3. Enjoy as soon as it has cooled just enough to dip a finger into.

4. Can be stored refrigerated in an airtight container for up to a week—mix well and heat gently before use.

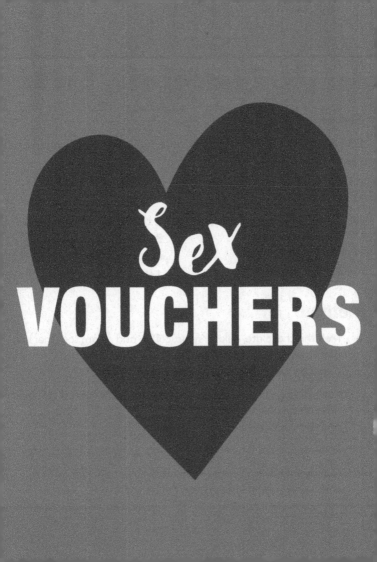

To . . . .

I PROMISE...

...to cook you dinner wearing nothing but an apron.

Signed. . . . .

Date. . . . .

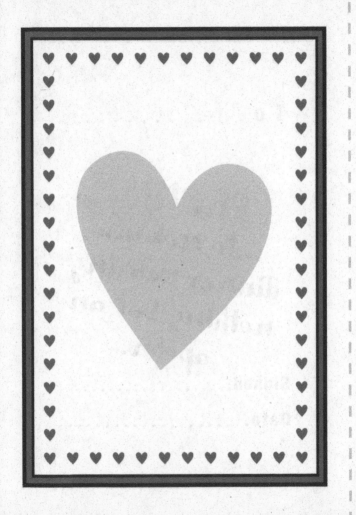

To. . . . . , . . .

I PROMISE...

...to fulfil your every sexual demand for a whole day.

Signed. . . . .

Date. . . . .

To . . . .

I PROMISE...

...to send you juicy text messages describing your hottest desires while you're at work.

Signed . . . .

Date . . . .

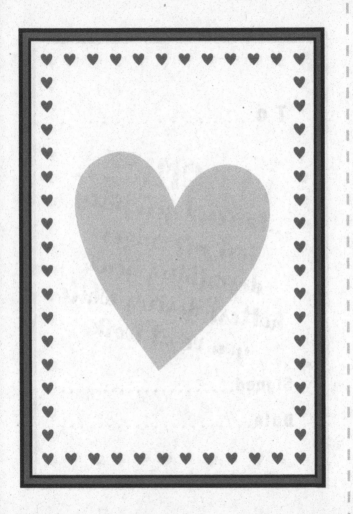

To . . . .

I PROMISE...

...to pleasure you
with your favorite
sex toy.

Signed . . . .

Date . . . .

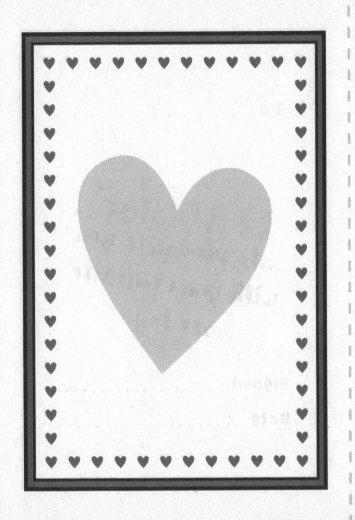

To . . . .

I PROMISE...
...to perform
a kinky dance
for you.

Signed . . . .

Date . . . .

To . . . .

I PROMISE...
...to lick every
inch of your
body.

Signed. . . . .

Date. . . . .

CONCLUSION

Thank you for being here for this journey through the cheeky, naughty and downright steamy. Hopefully you've picked up a few gems that will keep your sheets sizzling long after the final page is turned. Keep this book on your bedside table for whenever you need a bit of inspiration, and remember the two sexiest things of all: clear communication and confidence.

Have fun.

Stay safe.

Live, love, lust.

ANSWERS

Page 90

```
U K W J O B T S U A J N P A T
S P C E M I U K A P G Q W V G
H H L A P M Z M S R V K W A
J A O F B N M N M S C H W A
X J B U V R Y U P E W I U F G
T X M F I M E F Y H G W N U
Y P I W O D B T U T S L C L
K V Q K Z U E D O W U O S R
P X G A T R T R R L O U M L X
R U C T N I P P L E M V L Q I
V Y Q K B M C W E B Q Q K J B
B C C T B B Y H A L W Q N X Y
N L B V L L R B Q I S R R N V
Z S X R A E F Q W E F U Z N X
```

Pages 92-93

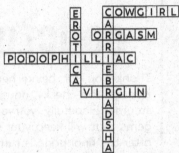

Page 94

Path 3 leads to the nipple.

Page 91

Word ladder

One possible solution:

give → hive → hire → here → herd → head

Anagrams: Deep Throat, The Devil in Miss Jones, Flesh Gordon

Page 95

```
X D I N E X H Y P L Z R W L B
A J N C G G D C K Q O W G L
D J N S E U S S I T W U N O
E V R I O D Z D A Z L R L E N
H S F C R B Y R D P K L E G D
S L O S F R B F L V X E J A F
C M U K L A X R T G Q S O
L L Q U V E N K E A X S A D
P V B D H A N D C U F F S A D
W E Y W H K E I Z L U Y G M F
P H M C I Q J F H F A W P K H
Z U W G B K Z N Z I W M P G F
F E F R S L I Y A J S J R M D
E K K Z I G C Z O V L I T S V
H W X H Z V W P A Z L O P M O
```

Page 96

Word ladder

One possible solution: pull→
bull → bulk → sulk → suck

Anagrams: cunnilingus,
fellatio, penetration

Page 97

Path 2 leads to the lolly.

Pages 98-99

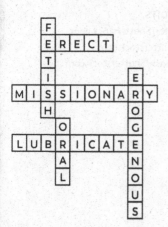

Page 100

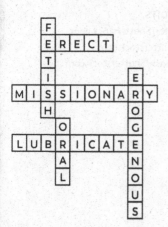

Page 101

Word ladder

One possible solution:
moan → morn → corn →
core → come

Anagrams: The sixty-nine,
Missionary, Doggy style

IMAGE CREDITS
Hand and foot icons © Rvector/Shutterstock.com
Ice lollies © tandaV/Shutterstock.com
Rose and heart icons © Bibadash/Shutterstock.com